MW01483136

Sophia's Story

A Young Girl's Battle With Childhood Cancer

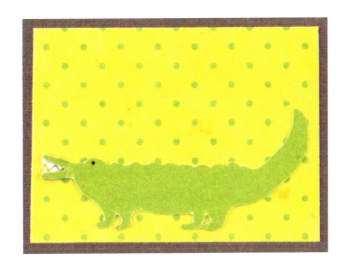

Tessie Goheen

Published by:

Square Publishing
P.O. Box D
Indianola, WA 98342
square.publishing@gmail.com

Distributed by:

EDK Distribution, LLC
edkbookdistribution.com
(206) 227-8179

Text and Illustrations Copyright © 2014 by Tessie Goheen

All rights reserved. No part of this book may be reproduced, stored in, or introduced into a retrieval system, or transmitted in any form, or by any means (electronic, mechanical, photocopying, recording, or otherwise) without the prior written permission of the publisher.

10 9 8 7 6 5 4 3 2 1

Printed in the United States of America

LCCN 2014908754
ISBN 978-0-9832635-5-5

Design: Leigh Faulkner
Photography: Amie Hancock

This book is dedicated to:

Mom, Katie, and Becky. Without your love and support, this book would not have been possible. Thank you for everything you do for me.

To Josiah, Elijah, and Andrew. You bring me so much happiness.

I love you all so much.

Thank you to:

Taryn Oestreich, you saw the potential of this book even before I did.

Erik & Leigh, thank you for making this book possible.

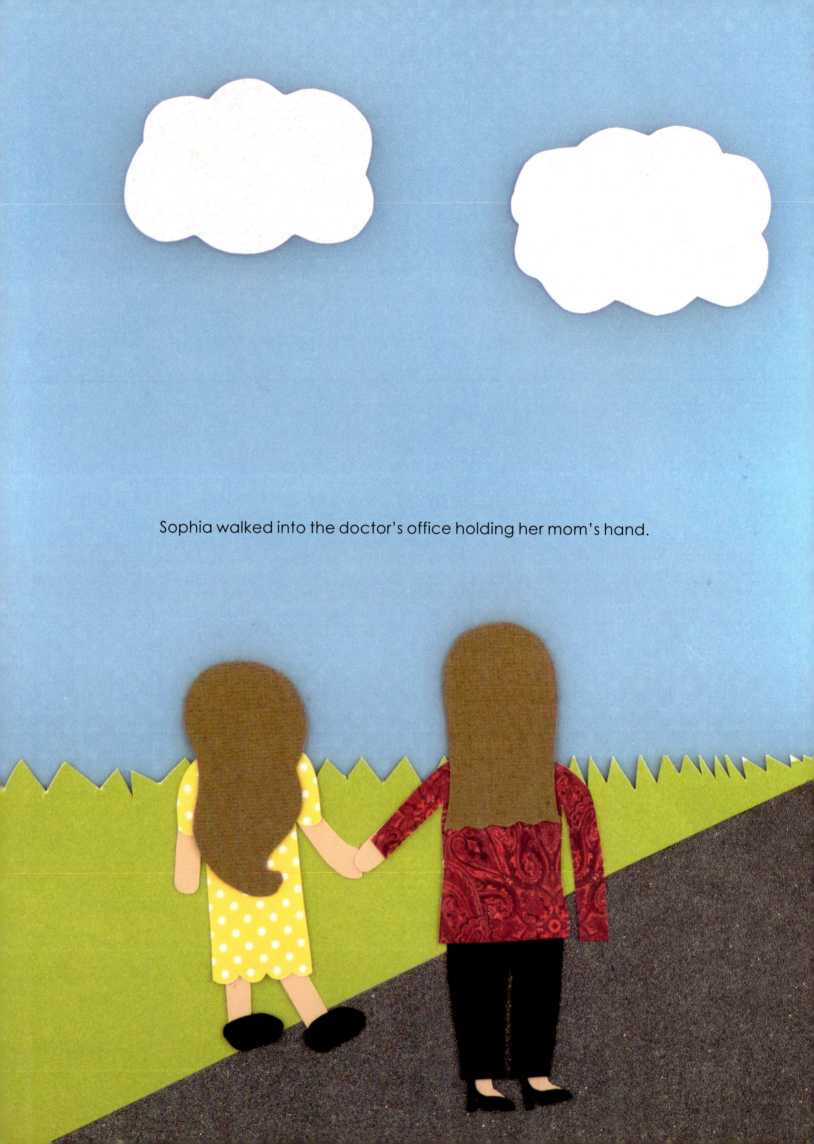

Sophia walked into the doctor's office holding her mom's hand.

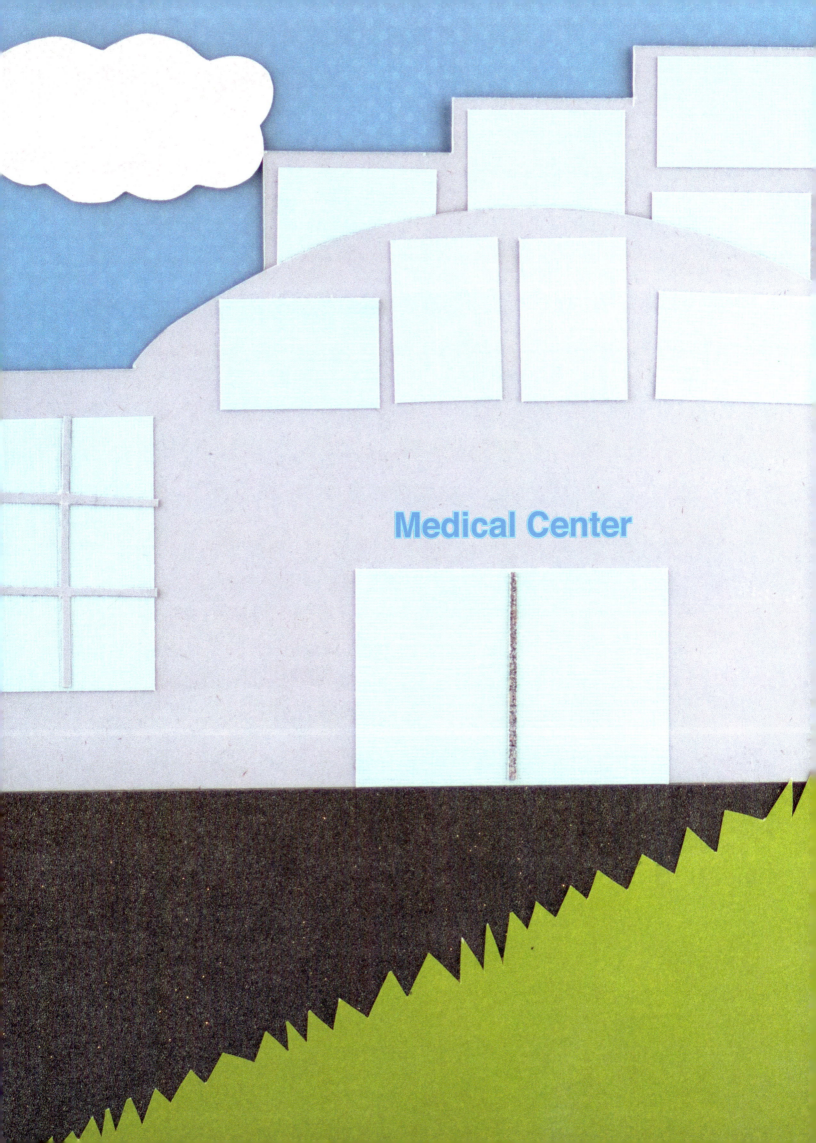

Medical Center

The nurse led Sophia and her mom back to the exam room. "Sophia, you can take a seat on the exam table. What brings you in today?" asked the nurse.

"I have a bump," said Sophia.

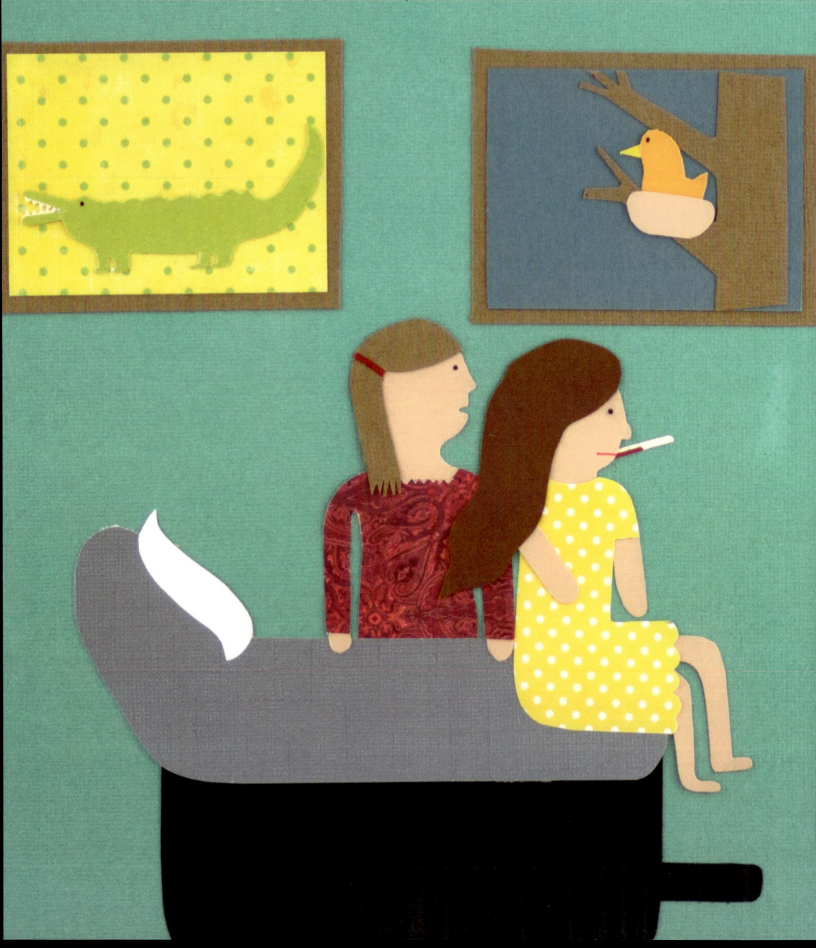

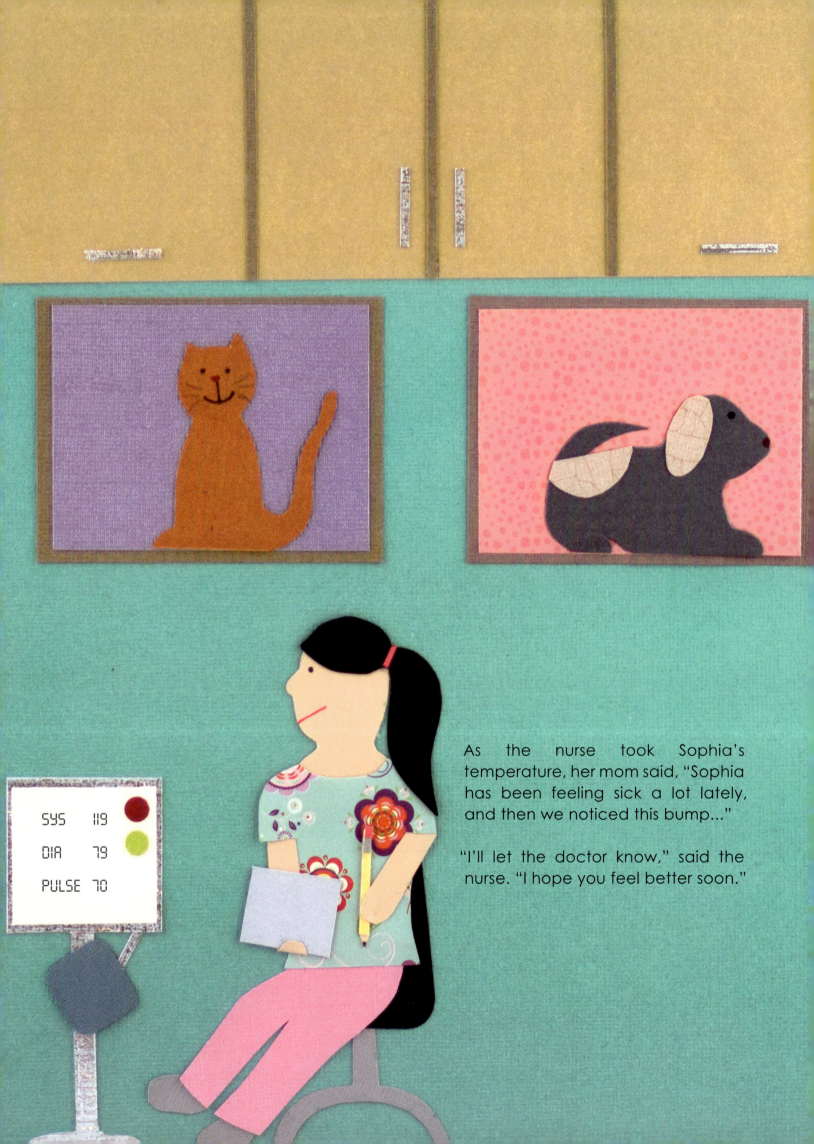

As the nurse took Sophia's temperature, her mom said, "Sophia has been feeling sick a lot lately, and then we noticed this bump..."

"I'll let the doctor know," said the nurse. "I hope you feel better soon."

SYS 119
DIA 79
PULSE 70

The doctor came in soon after the nurse left. She looked inside Sophia's mouth, ears, and nose. She felt along the side of her face and behind her ears. She listened to her heart and lungs. Then she looked at her arms, legs, and back. "Can you show me where your bump is Sophia?"

"It's right here on my stomach," Sophia answered.

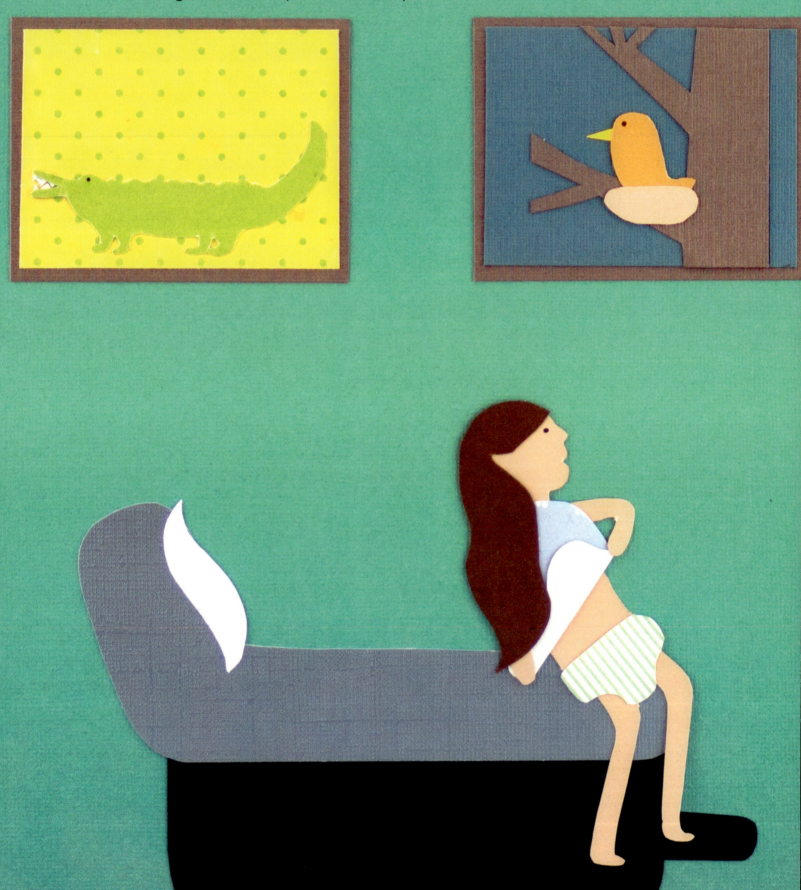

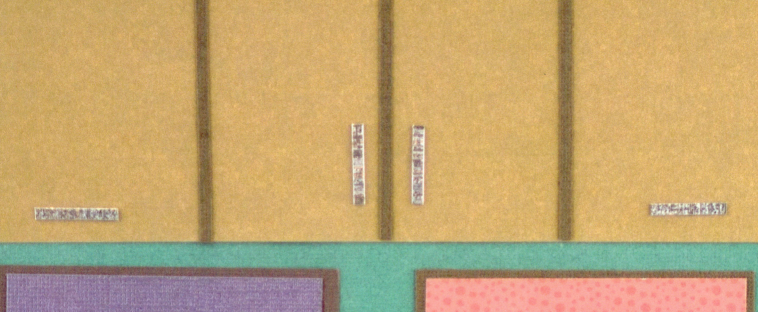

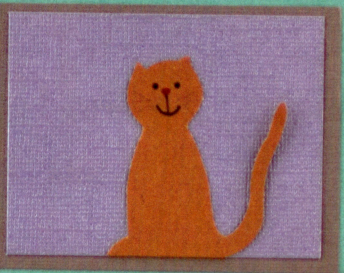

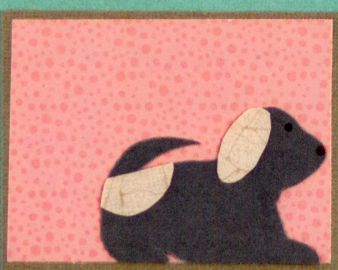

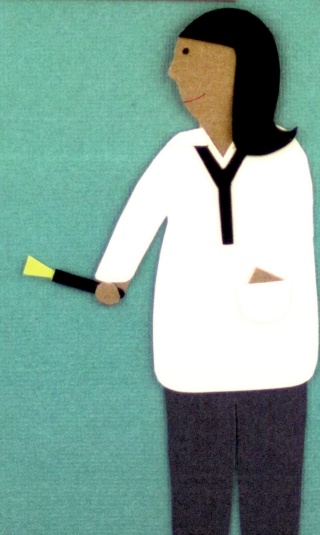

"Sophia, I'm going to send you to the lab. At the lab they will draw some blood from your arm."

"What do you mean draw blood?" asked Sophia.

"Drawing blood is just another way of saying a nurse will use a small needle to take some blood out of your arm. It may help us figure out what's making you feel so bad."

Sophia was scared about getting her blood drawn, but her mom promised to stay with her the whole time. When they reached the end of the hallway, Sophia grabbed her mom's hand and squeezed tight. Sophia read a book while she waited for her turn.

"Number 26!" called the man working in the lab. Sophia was number 26. She grabbed her mom's hand again as she walked into the lab.

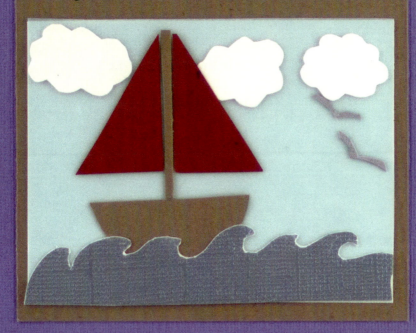

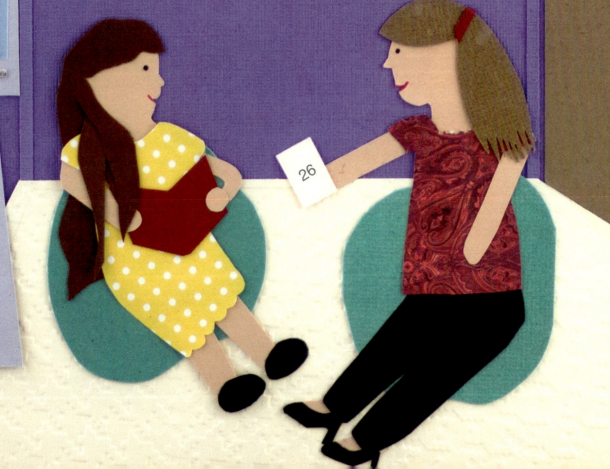

Please
Take a
Number

27

26

LAB

"Nice to meet you Sophia, my name is Andrew. I'm what they call a phlebotomist, meaning I'm someone trained to draw blood. You can sit down right here, and your mom can stand next to you and hold your hand." The phlebotomist tied a string around her arm, kind of like a rubber band, and gave Sophia a ball to squeeze. It didn't take very long, and when she was done the phlebotomist gave her a band-aid and a sticker. "You did great, and you were so brave. Take care, Sophia."

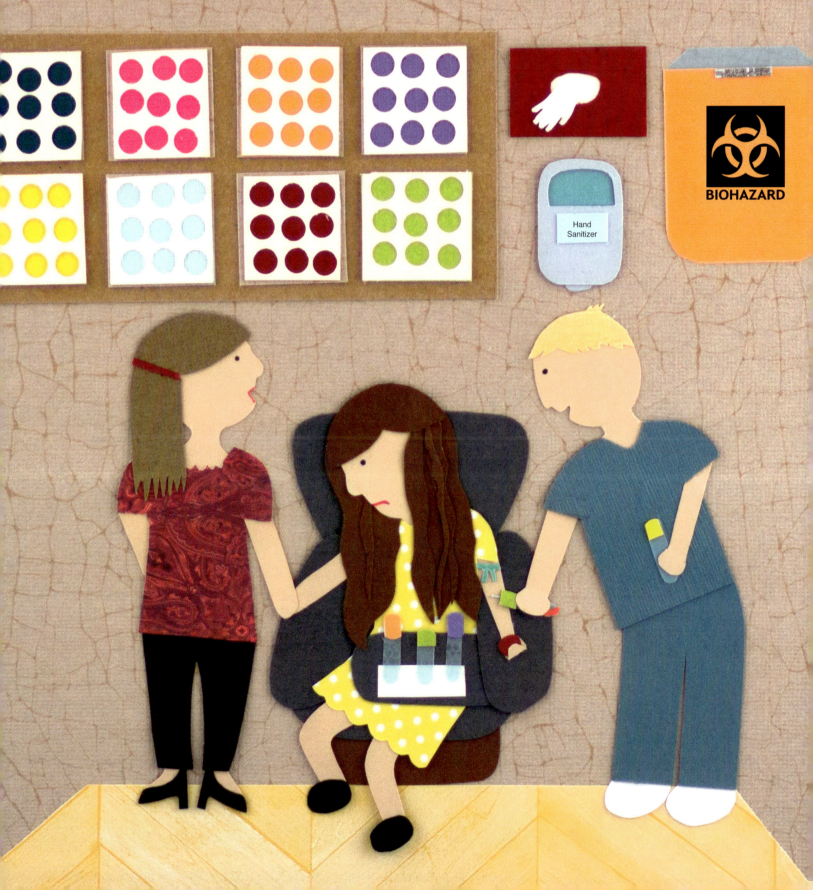

The next day, Sophia's mom got a phone call from the doctor. She wanted Sophia to come back in to have a biopsy. A biopsy is when they take out small samples of skin or tissue to see whether or not it contains a disease. Sophia could tell her mom was nervous — she was feeling nervous too.

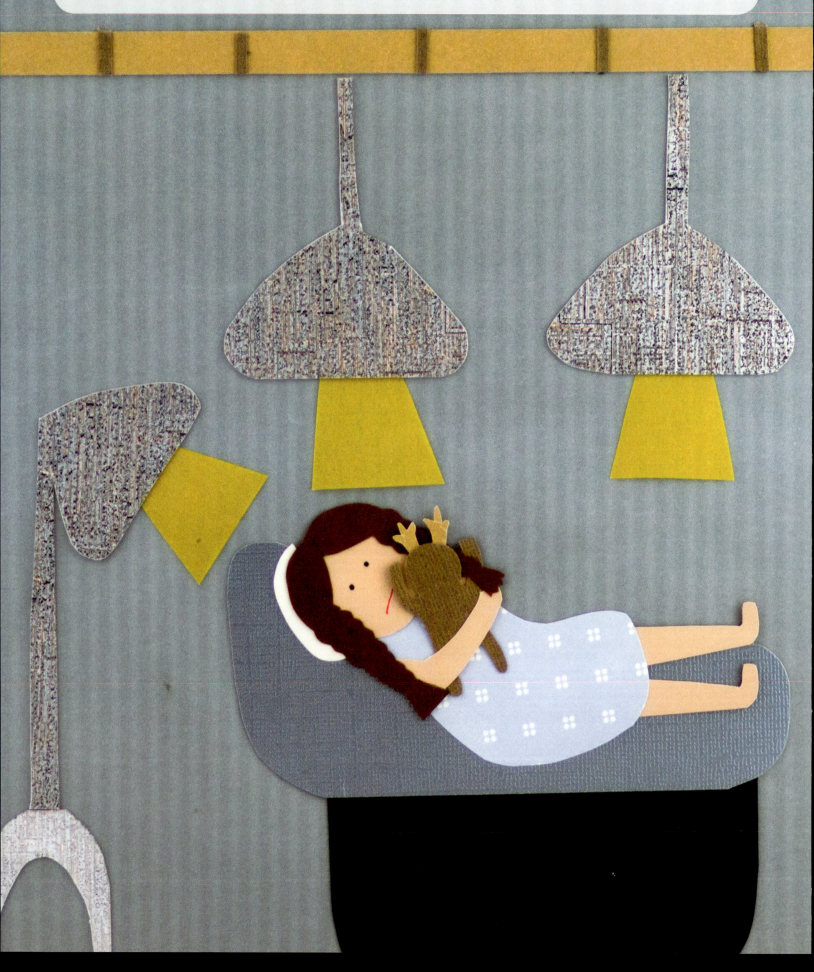

Her mom explained to her that the doctors would numb the biopsy area so she wouldn't be able to feel anything. Then the doctors would use a hollow needle to take out a small piece of her bump. Afterwards, they would send the sample to a lab. The scientists at the lab would examine the sample to see if it had any abnormal cells.

On the way home, Sophia's mom stopped for ice cream, Sophia's favorite. She explained that the results of the biopsy take a few days to get back.

"Don't worry, Sophia," her mom said. "Everything will be okay."

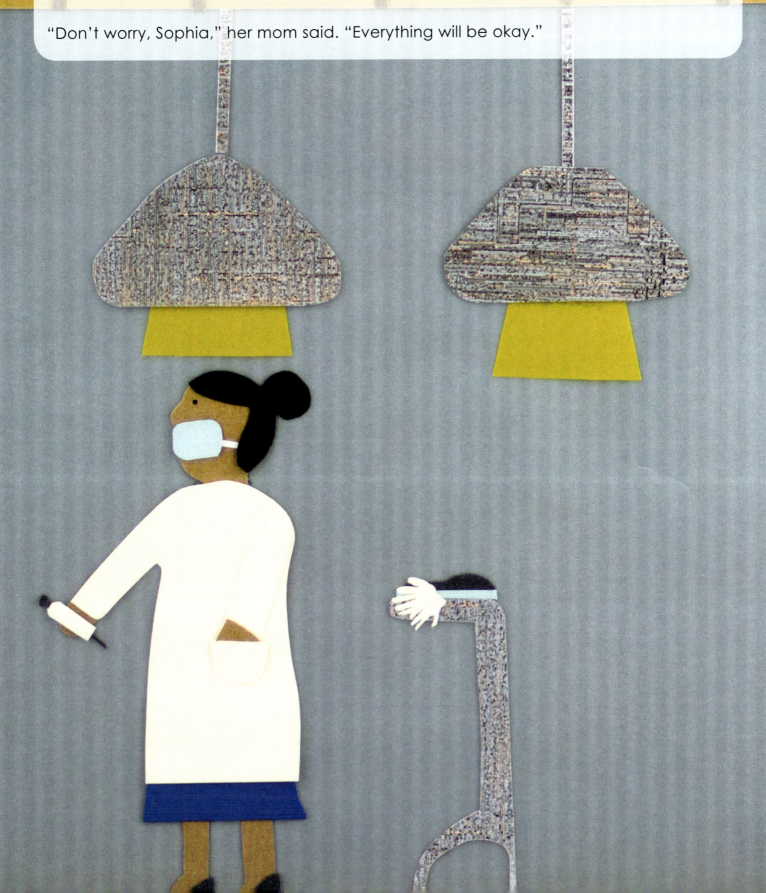

When Sophia got home from school on Monday, her mom told her that she had cancer. Sophia had heard of cancer. She knew that it made people very sick, but she felt okay, just a little tired. How could she have cancer?

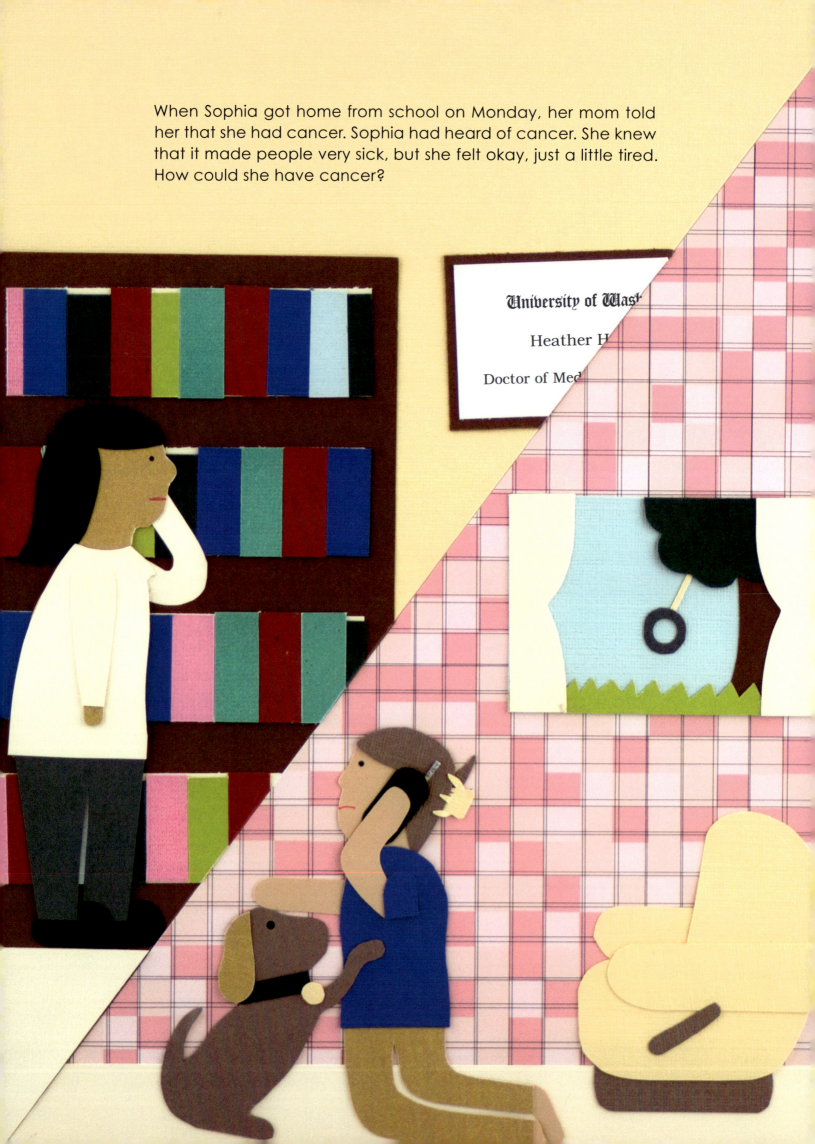

"Sophia, next Wednesday, we will be going to see a new doctor. This doctor is called an oncologist. An oncologist is a doctor that specializes in cancer." Her mom began to cry as she wrapped Sophia into a big hug. Sophia was scared, but she felt safe knowing her mom would always be there.

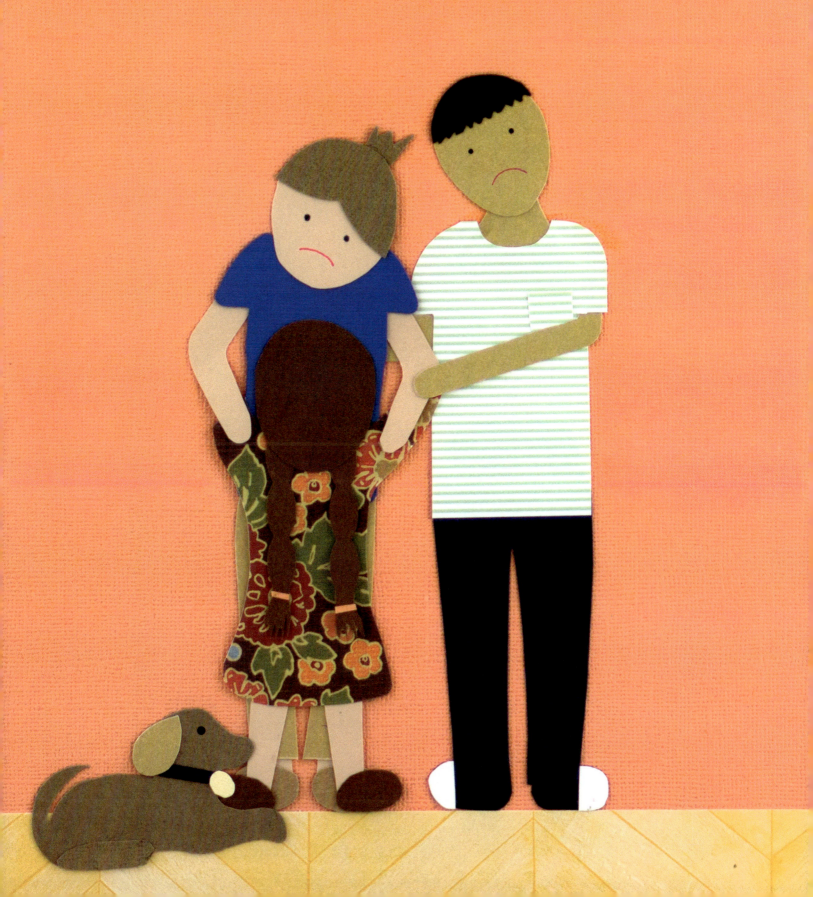

Wednesday came fast, and soon Sophia was in the car with her mom driving toward the hospital. When they arrived, Sophia's mom took her to check in. After a few minutes, a doctor came out of the back room.

"Hi, Sophia. You can call me Dr. Ron," he said.

Dr. Ron took Sophia back to an exam room. In the exam room, Dr. Ron sat down. "Sophia, I want to tell you about this disease and answer any questions you have.

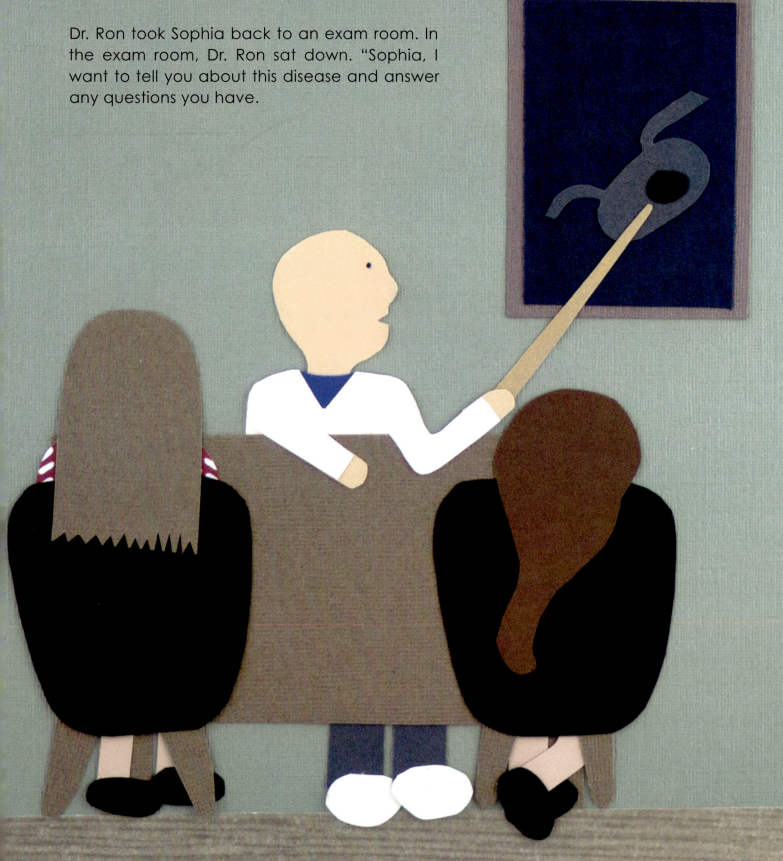

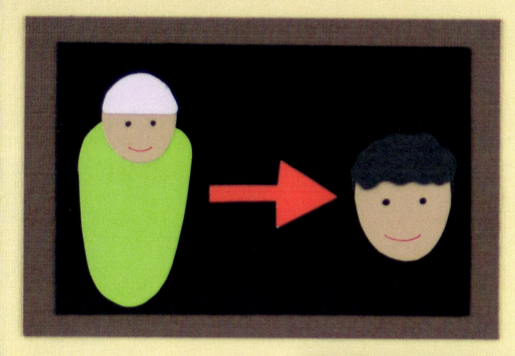

"Sophia, you have what we call a sarcoma. This means that your cancer developed in the tissue of your body. However, cancer can develop in virtually any part of your body at any age. So, while your cancer is in your stomach, someone else could have cancer in their bones or even their brain. Cancer can spread through your blood or even your lymph nodes."

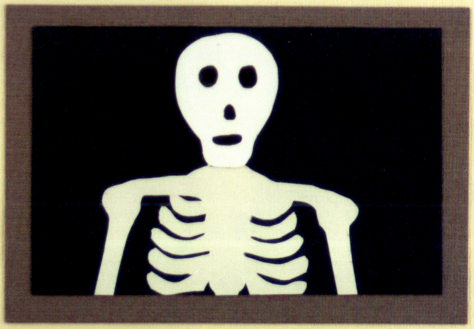

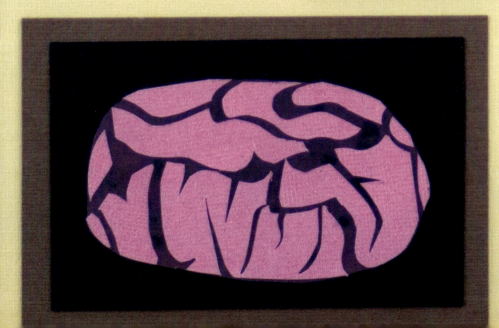

"I still don't really understand what cancer is," said Sophia.

Dr. Ron drew a picture as he explained. "Usually when your cells divide, if a cell becomes damaged, it does not divide any further. The damaged cell dies."

"Cancer cells are different. The damaged cell keeps dividing. Cancer is a disease that happens when the cells in your body grow and divide uncontrollably. The cells grow and divide so fast that they invade your body and spread."

Cell Division

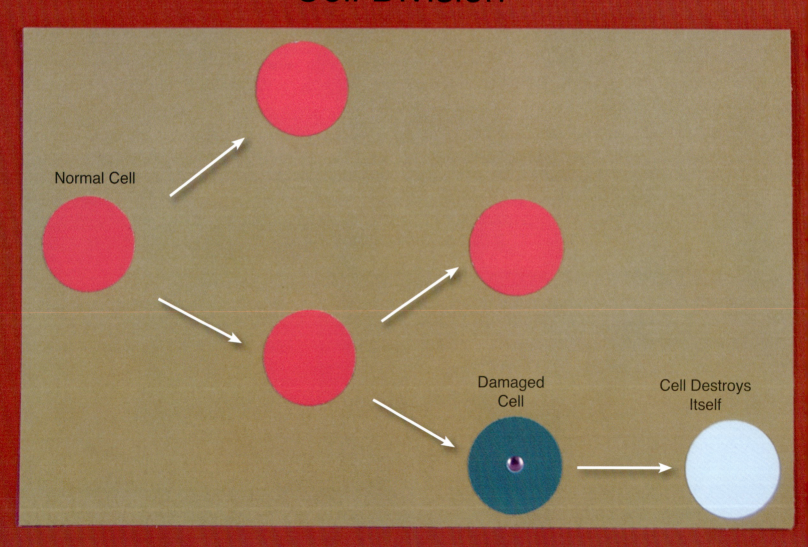

Normal Cell

Damaged Cell

Cell Destroys Itself

Cancer Cell Division

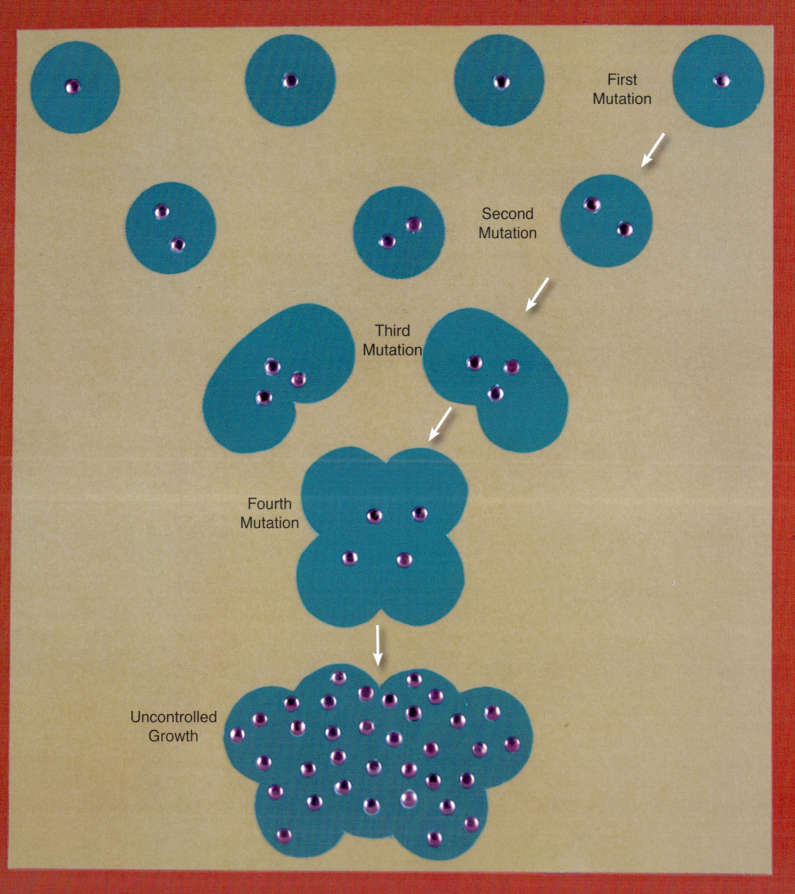

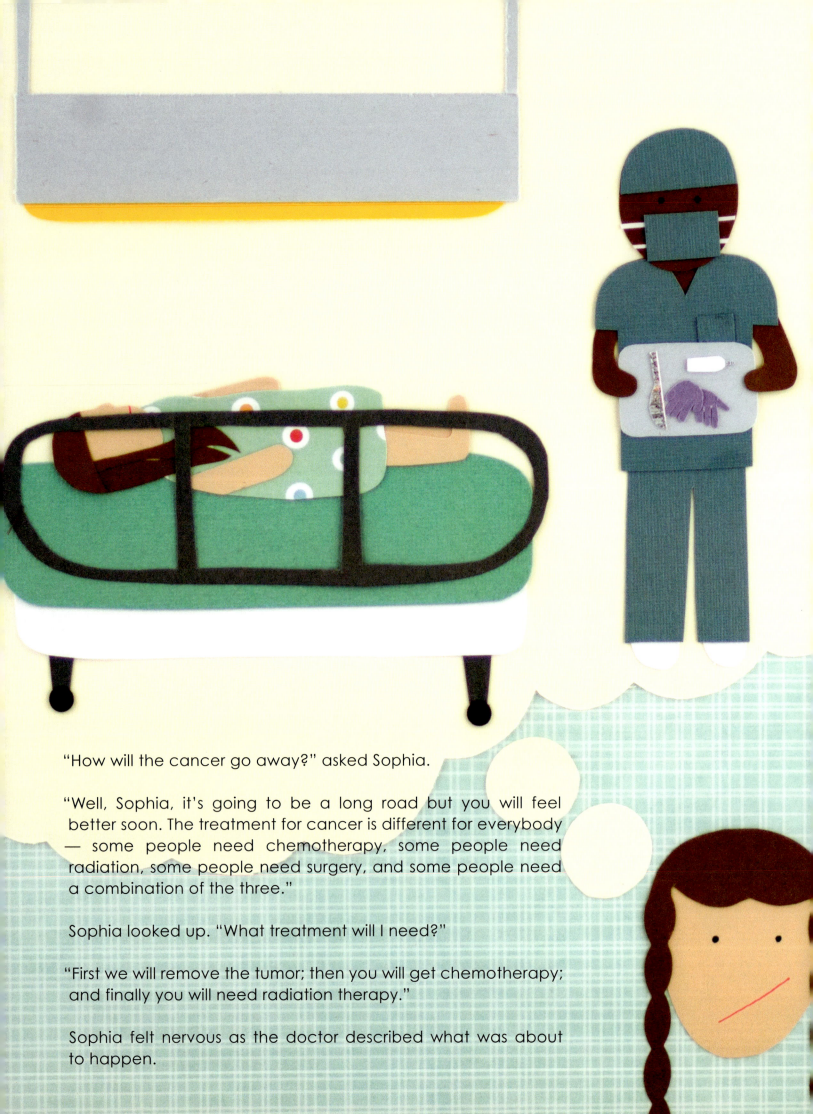

"How will the cancer go away?" asked Sophia.

"Well, Sophia, it's going to be a long road but you will feel better soon. The treatment for cancer is different for everybody — some people need chemotherapy, some people need radiation, some people need surgery, and some people need a combination of the three."

Sophia looked up. "What treatment will I need?"

"First we will remove the tumor; then you will get chemotherapy; and finally you will need radiation therapy."

Sophia felt nervous as the doctor described what was about to happen.

"When you go in for surgery, your mom can stay with you until you go back into the operating room. Then a nurse will stay with you and give you some medicine that makes you very tired. After you fall asleep, the doctor will start the surgery to remove the tumor. You won't feel anything while you are sleeping. When you wake up, your mom will be there waiting for you and you might feel sore. You'll stay here in the hospital until you feel better."

"When you go in for surgery, you will likely get a port put in your body. The port goes in right under your skin and is located below your collar bone."

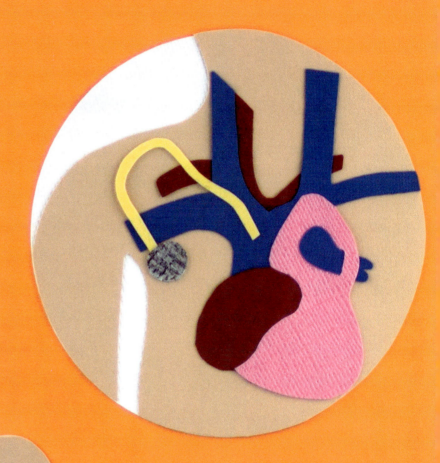

Portacath

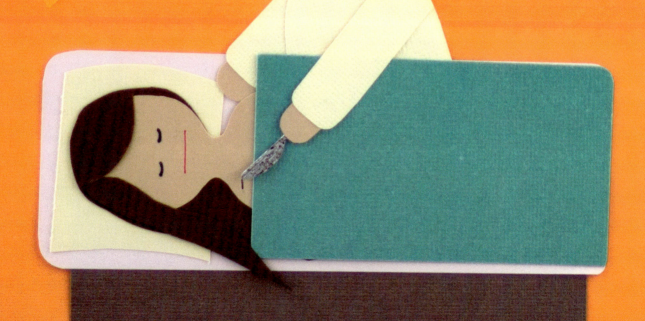

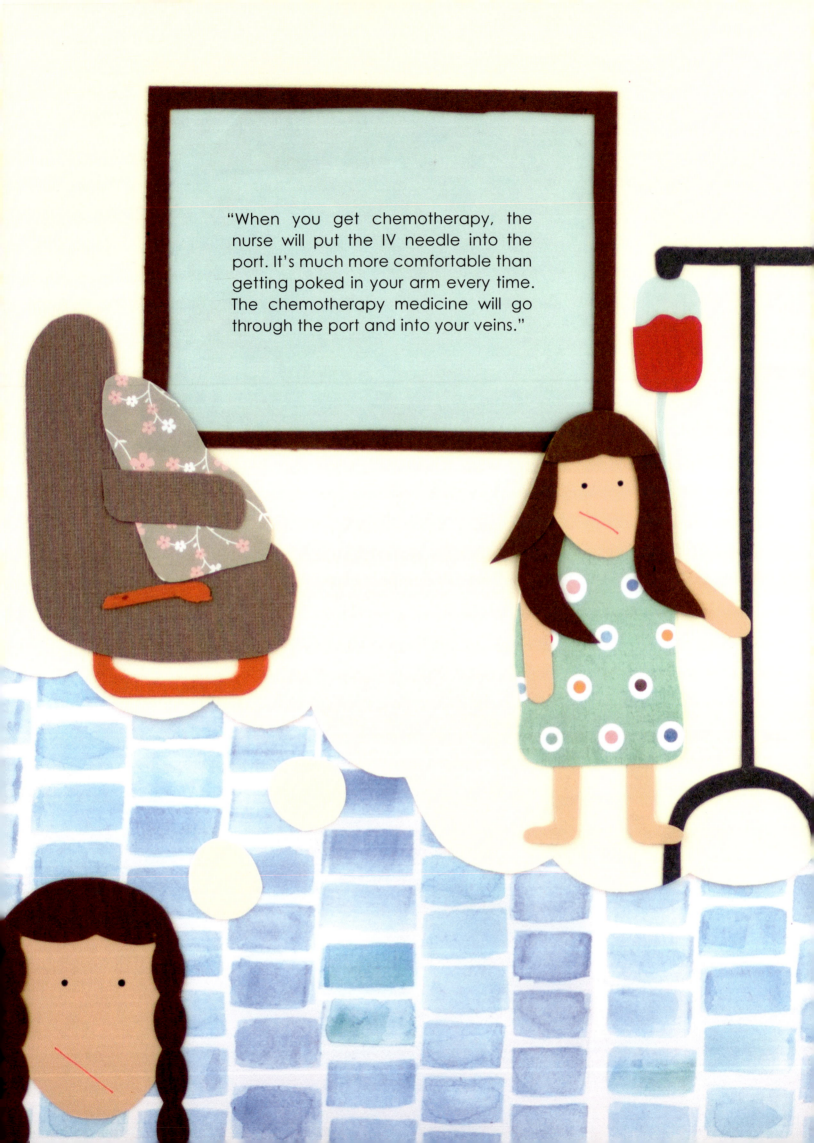

"When you get chemotherapy, the nurse will put the IV needle into the port. It's much more comfortable than getting poked in your arm every time. The chemotherapy medicine will go through the port and into your veins."

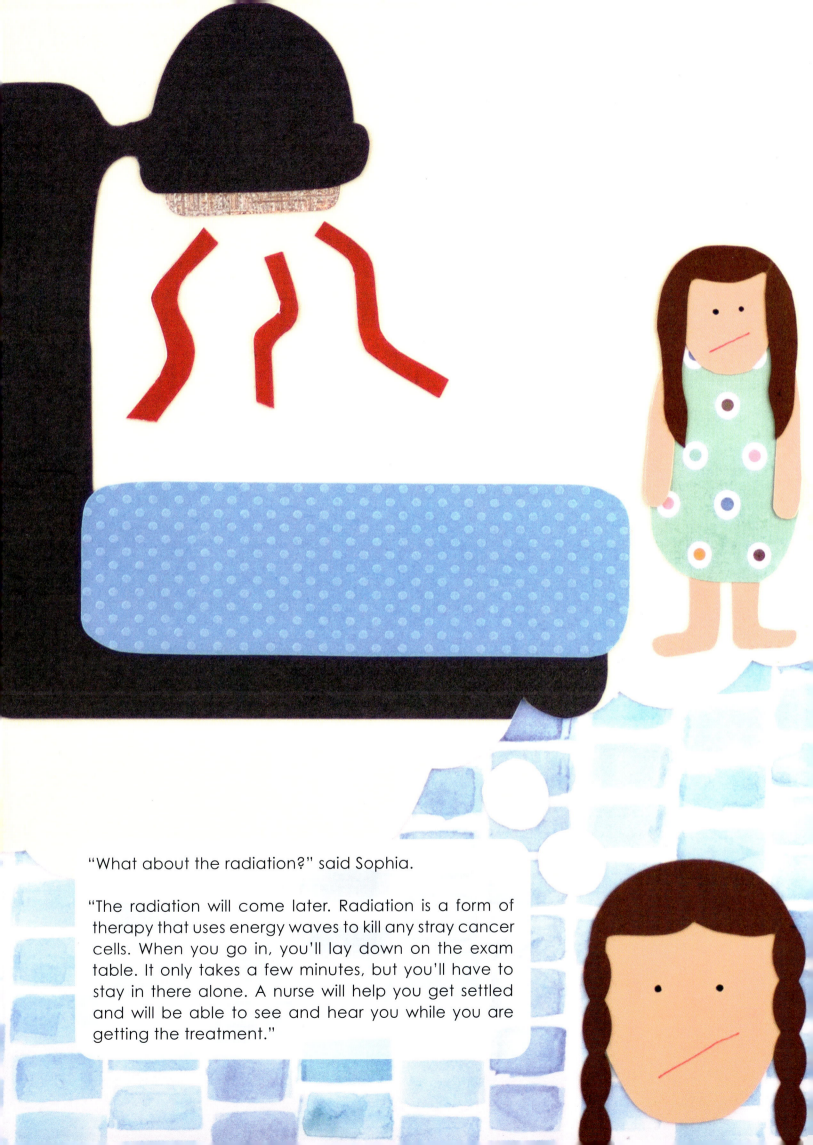

"What about the radiation?" said Sophia.

"The radiation will come later. Radiation is a form of therapy that uses energy waves to kill any stray cancer cells. When you go in, you'll lay down on the exam table. It only takes a few minutes, but you'll have to stay in there alone. A nurse will help you get settled and will be able to see and hear you while you are getting the treatment."

"Your chemotherapy will be given to you here at the hospital, and for this treatment, your mom or dad will be able to stay with you the whole time. Chemotherapy is medicine that goes in through an IV and kills rapidly dividing cells."

"You mean it kills cancer," said Sophia.

"Yes," said Dr. Ron, "but it can also harm other cells that divide quickly. I'll tell you more about that soon.

"Remember when I told you that the chemotherapy can harm other cells too?"

"Yes," said Sophia.

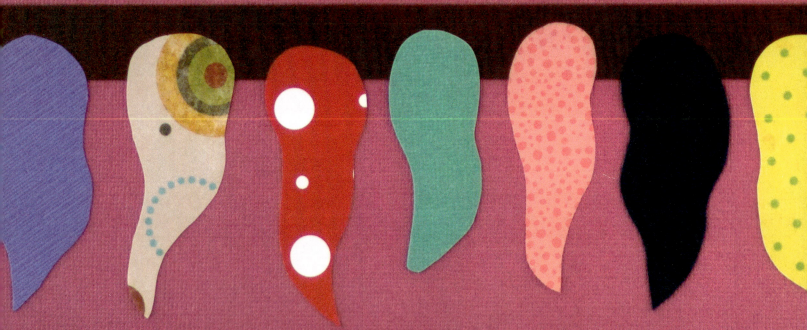

"Well, there are some side effects that come along with the chemotherapy. Chemotherapy can make you feel very sick. It can upset your stomach, make you feel very tired, and can even cause you to lose your hair."

Sophia couldn't imagine losing her hair. "I don't want to lose my hair!" she exclaimed.

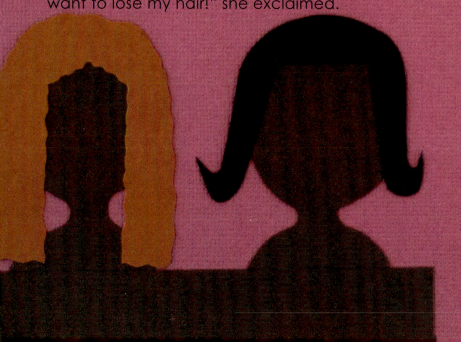
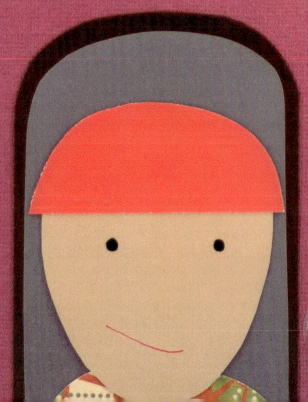

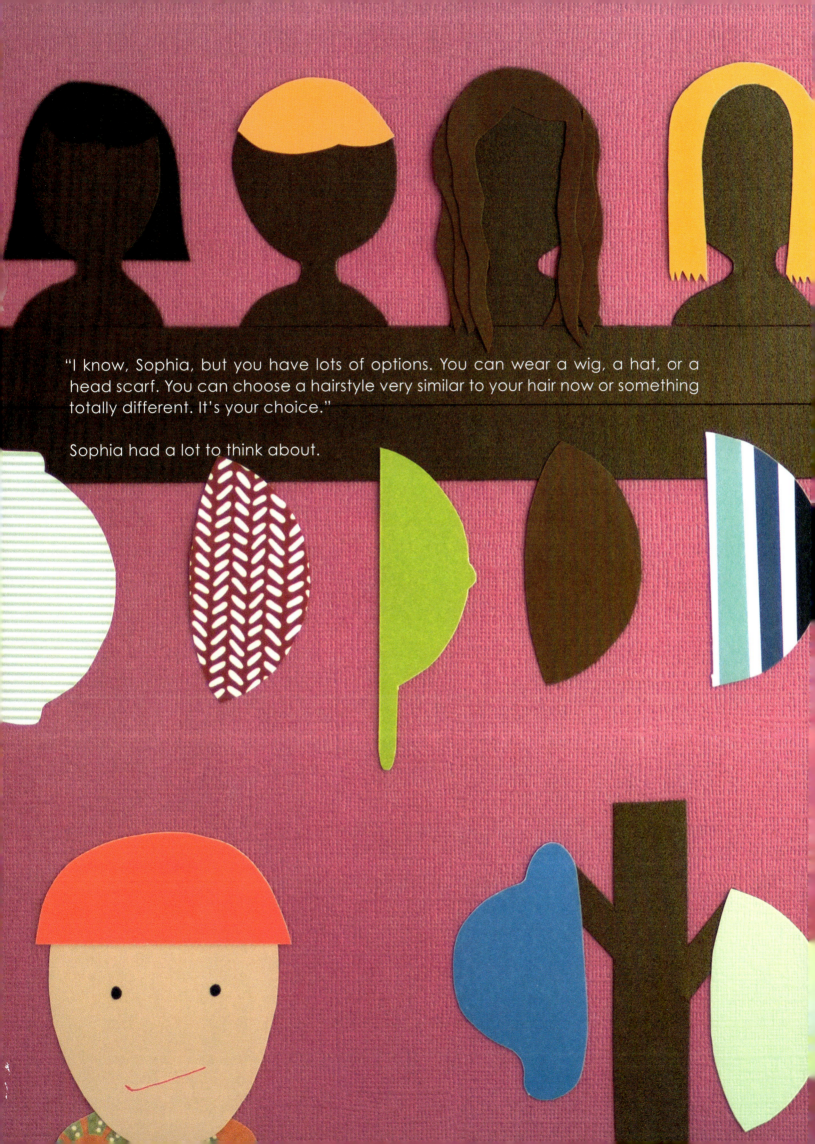

"I know, Sophia, but you have lots of options. You can wear a wig, a hat, or a head scarf. You can choose a hairstyle very similar to your hair now or something totally different. It's your choice."

Sophia had a lot to think about.

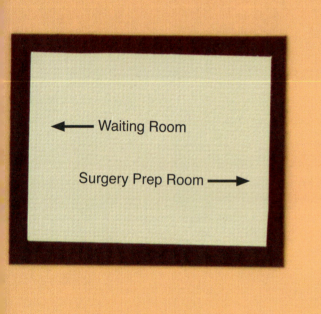

Waiting Room ←

Surgery Prep Room →

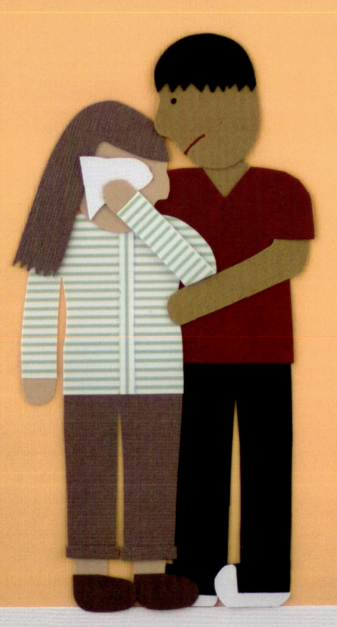

One week later, Sophia was back at the hospital ready for surgery. Her mom held her hand just like she did a couple of short weeks ago. When she went back for surgery Sophia hugged her special moose, JoJo.

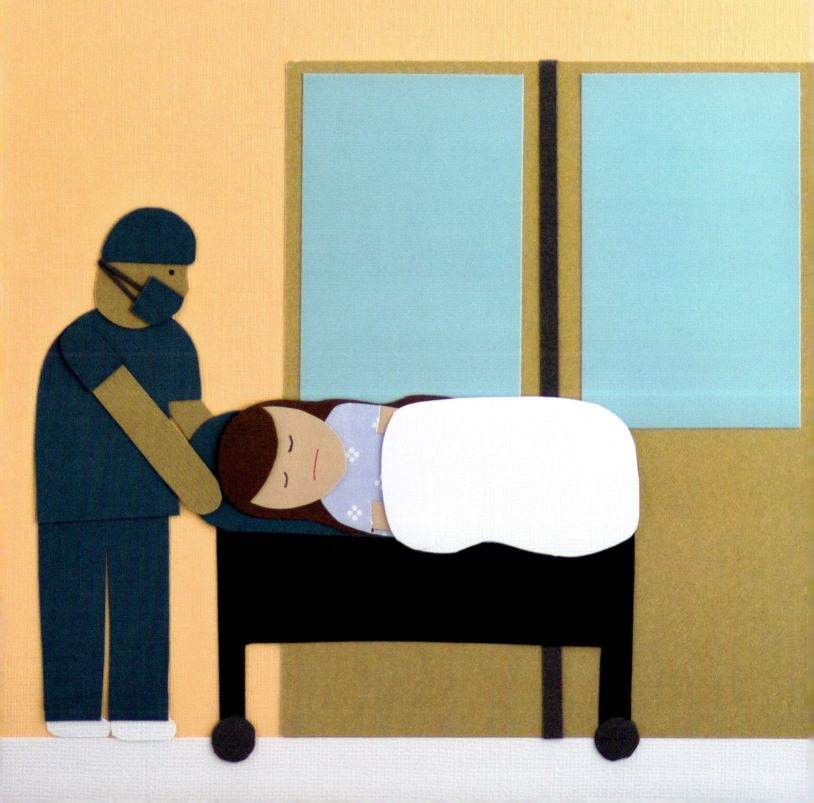

Just like Dr. Ron said, her mom was there when she woke up and was able to stay with her in the hospital, but Sophia still missed home.

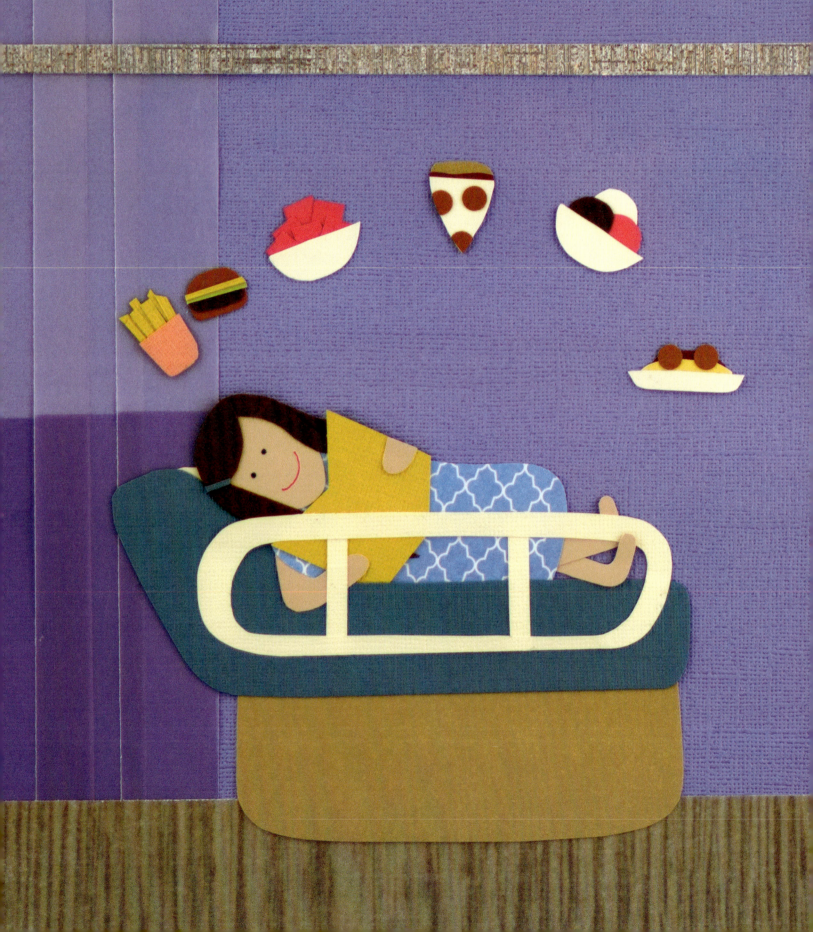

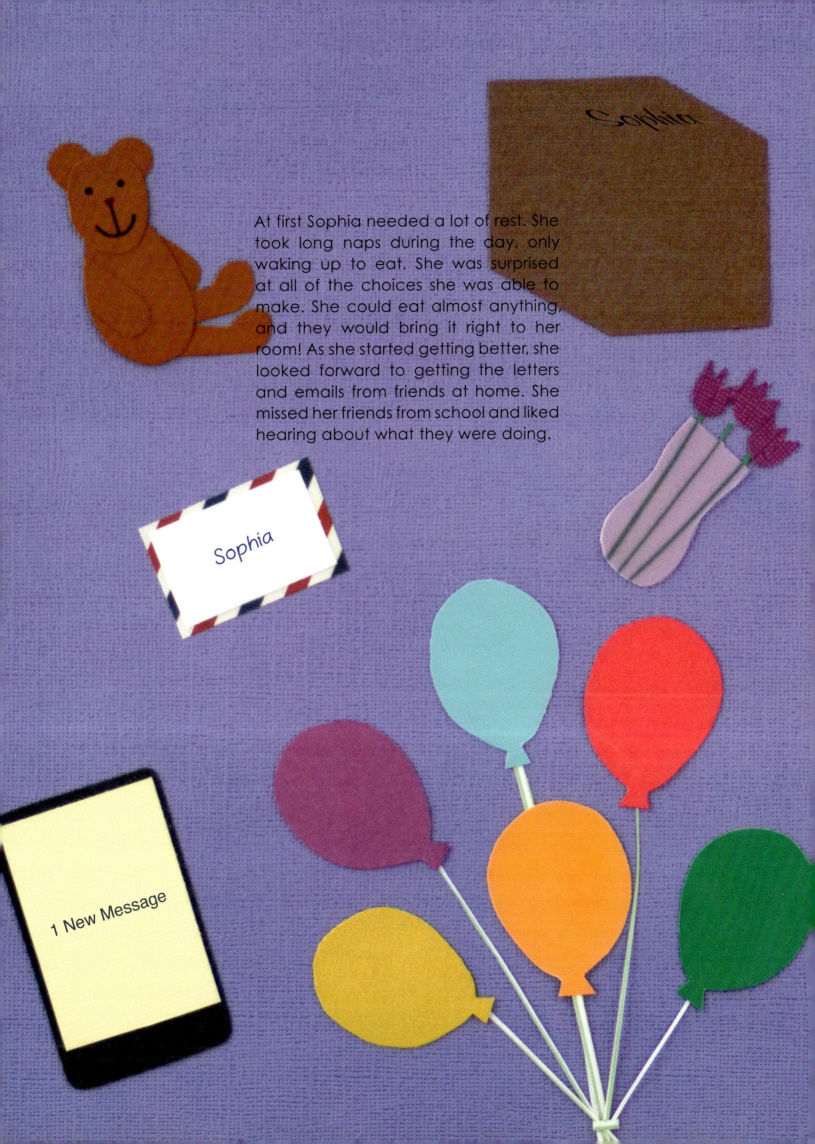

At first Sophia needed a lot of rest. She took long naps during the day, only waking up to eat. She was surprised at all of the choices she was able to make. She could eat almost anything, and they would bring it right to her room! As she started getting better, she looked forward to getting the letters and emails from friends at home. She missed her friends from school and liked hearing about what they were doing.

Sophia

Sophia

1 New Message

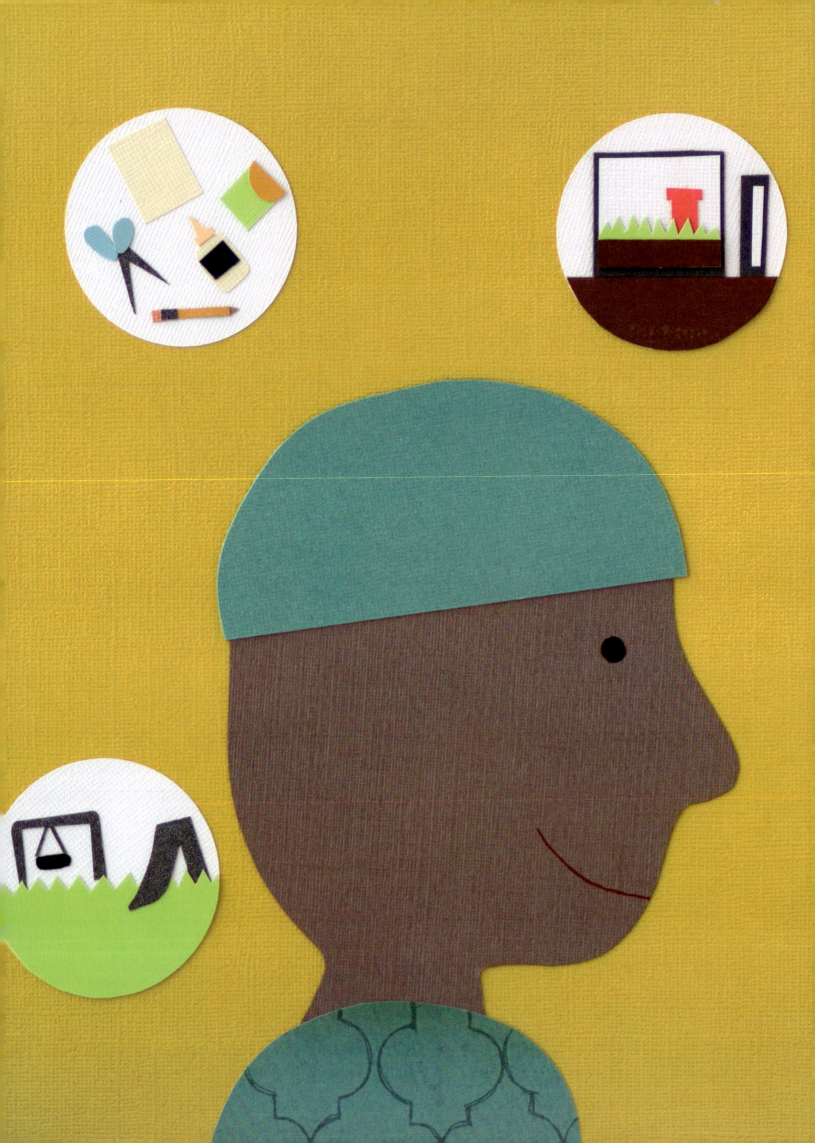

Sophia soon became friends with Addison, the girl she shared her hospital room with. Sophia liked talking with Addison, and it was fun to have someone to play with when she felt up to it. Even though Sophia didn't feel well, there were lots of things to do at the hospital. She missed home, but it wasn't so bad at the hospital. There were movies, games, and books. People came by to visit, and there were kind nurses that would check on her. There was even a teacher that came by to help her keep up with her work from school.

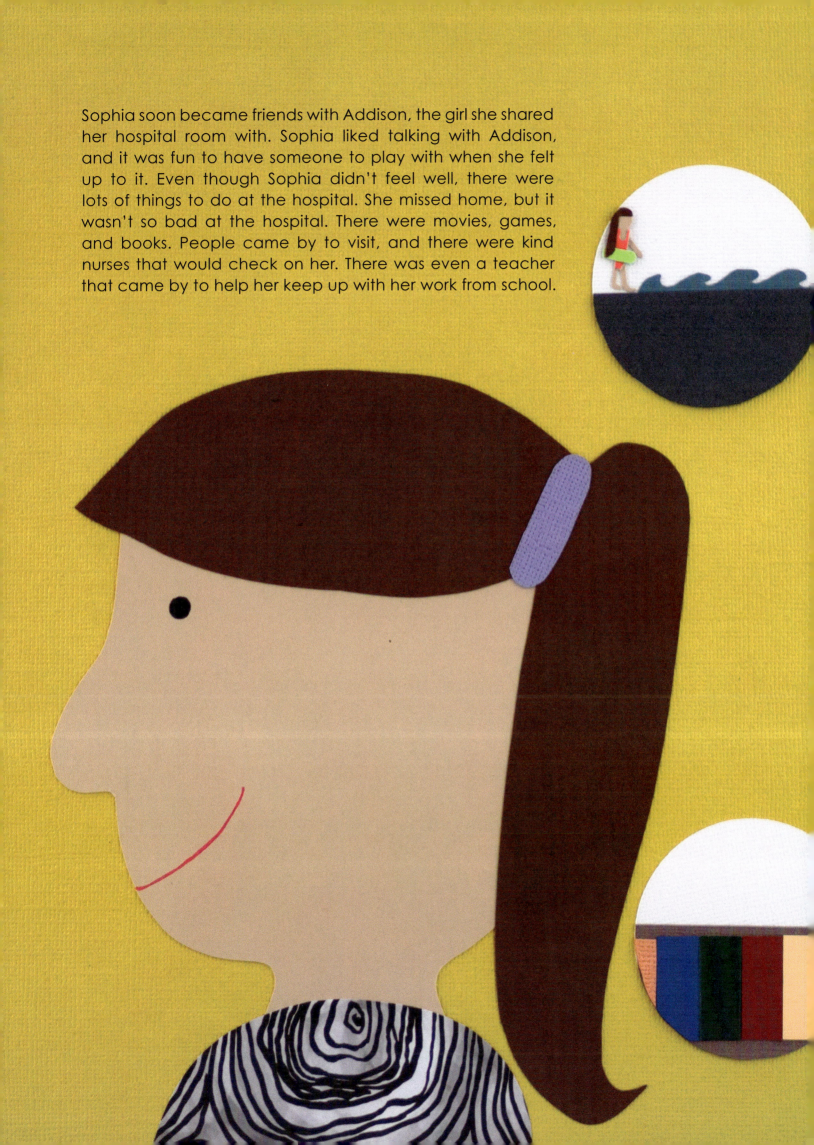

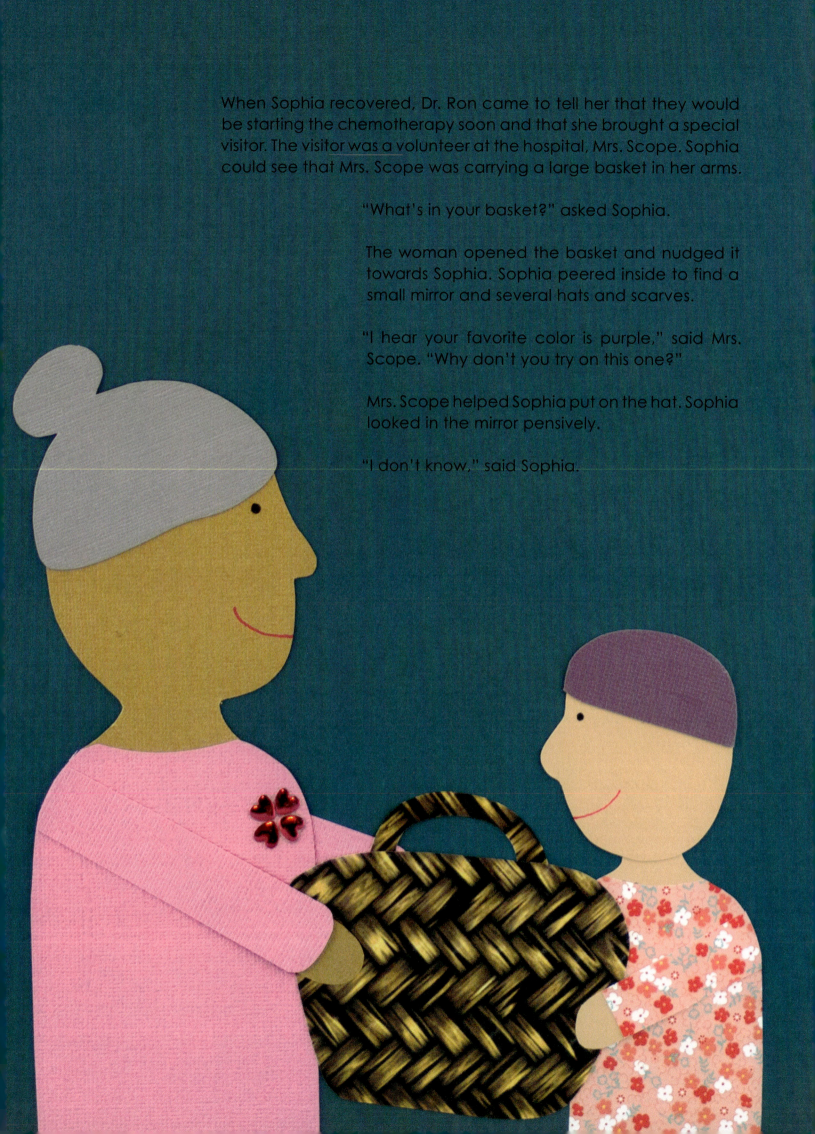

When Sophia recovered, Dr. Ron came to tell her that they would be starting the chemotherapy soon and that she brought a special visitor. The visitor was a volunteer at the hospital, Mrs. Scope. Sophia could see that Mrs. Scope was carrying a large basket in her arms.

"What's in your basket?" asked Sophia.

The woman opened the basket and nudged it towards Sophia. Sophia peered inside to find a small mirror and several hats and scarves.

"I hear your favorite color is purple," said Mrs. Scope. "Why don't you try on this one?"

Mrs. Scope helped Sophia put on the hat. Sophia looked in the mirror pensively.

"I don't know," said Sophia.

"I have an idea," said Mrs. Scope. She pulled out a pair of scissors from her bag and carefully clipped a small crocheted flower from her shirt. As she pinned it to the hat, she said, "You know Sophia, purple is my favorite color too — it's the color of hope."

Mrs. Scope gently placed the hat on Sophia's head. "Perfect!"

Sophia looked in the mirror; it was perfect. She still didn't want to lose her hair, but it was fun choosing new hats, and this purple hat was so special!

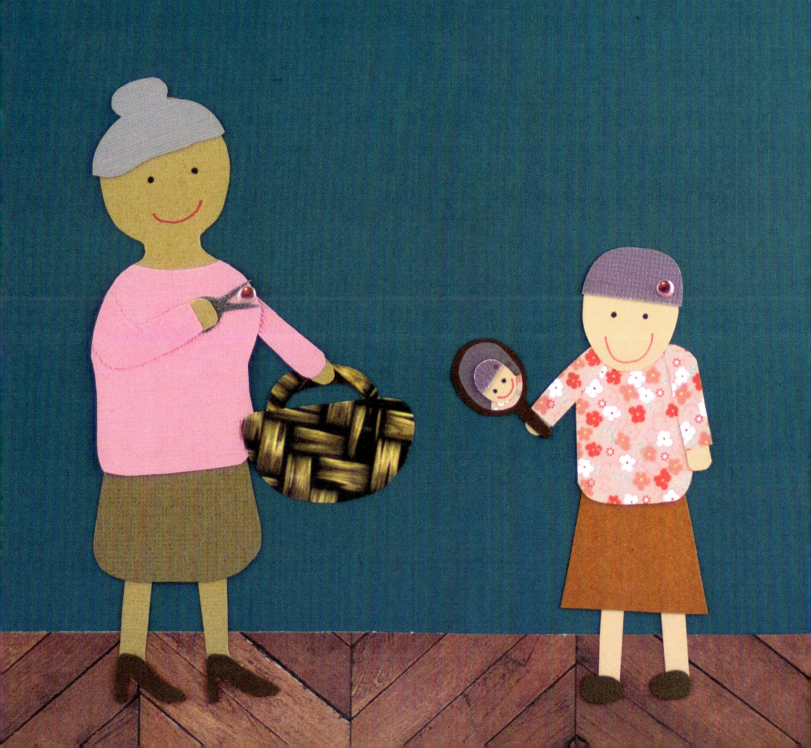

After several days of chemotherapy, Sophia was finally able to go home. She was tired and had to come back in two weeks for more chemotherapy, but she was happy to be able to go home.

As Sophia drove home with her mother, she thought about the last several weeks. She was proud of herself. She reached up and touched the flower on her hat. Even though it wasn't easy, she knew she would be okay.

Mrs. Scope was right; purple was the color of hope.

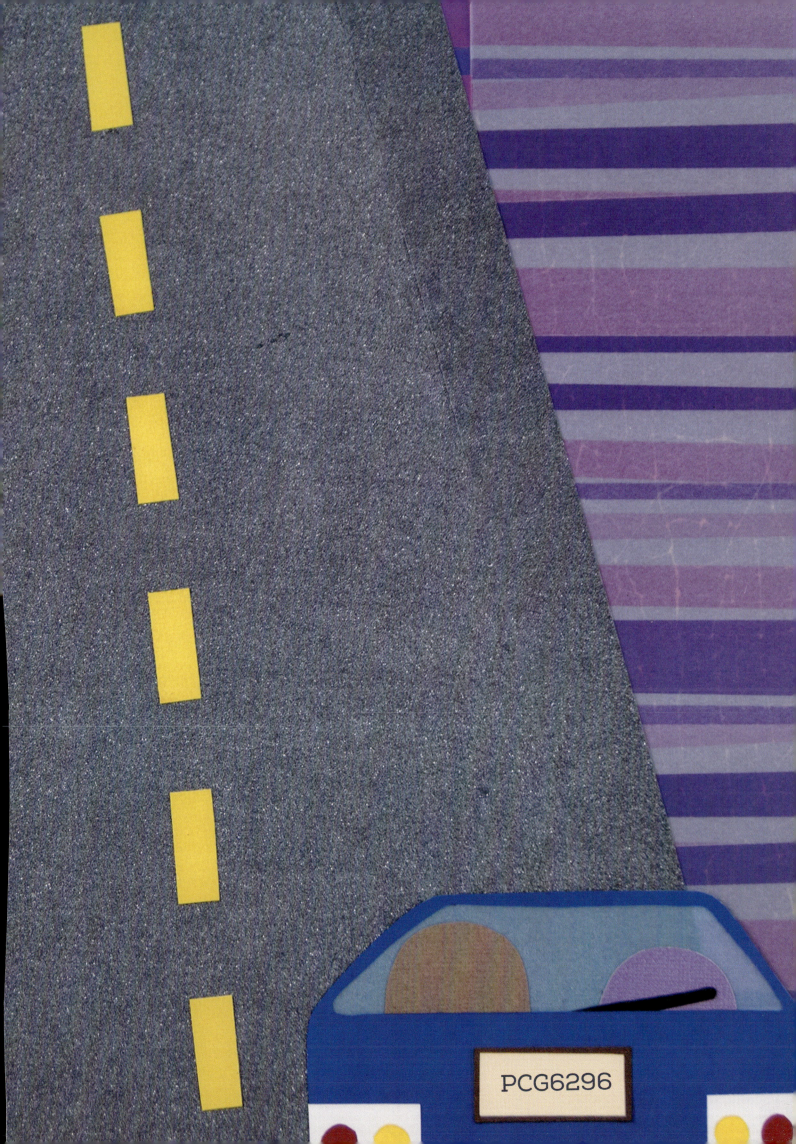

PCG6296